Organoid Intelligence

The Dawn of Living Machines

Mahdi Yousefian

2025

Published independently by Mahdi Yousefian

First Edition, 2025

Dedication

To my beloved parents, whose quiet strength and endless love

became the soil in which every thought of mine took root;

to my brother, a companion in both silence and laughter,

whose presence has been a lighthouse in uncertain seas;

and to the generations yet to come, who may inherit

not only our knowledge, but also our courage

to ask what lies beyond the horizon.

Preface

In the last two decades, the frontiers of science have witnessed an extraordinary convergence. Where once biology and computer science walked parallel roads, today they intertwine like the double helix itself — inseparable, interdependent, and fertile with possibility. Amidst this convergence, organoids have emerged not only as models of human biology, but as living testaments to the astonishing power of self-organization. They pulse, they signal, and in their silent choreography of cells, they reveal echoes of cognition itself.

The genesis of this book lay in a simple but unsettling question: what if the miniature worlds we nurture in the laboratory are not mere tools of science, but also windows into the essence of intelligence? This question grew into countless hours of reading, experimenting, and reflecting. It grew through dialogue — with mentors who reminded me that the heart of research lies not in answers but in questions; with colleagues whose critiques sharpened my vision; and with students whose raw curiosity reignited my own. Writing these chapters became less an act of scholarship and more an act of exploration.

The structure of the book reflects this vision. The opening chapters lay the biological foundations of organoid culture, exploring the self-organization of cells into three-dimensional tissues. From there, we move into protocols and technologies: the microelectrode arrays that capture electrical whispers, the molecular profiling tools that decode genetic symphonies, and the computational frameworks that turn signals into knowledge. Midway, the discussion widens to ethics, philosophy, and the dilemmas that haunt every scientific frontier: What constitutes consciousness? Where must society draw its lines? The final chapters turn resolutely toward the horizon — sketching futures in which organoids may serve as platforms for precision medicine, partners in artificial intelligence, or even co-authors of the human story.

Writing this book was as much a journey inward as it was outward. It demanded discipline, yet also surrender — for every attempt to control the narrative was met by the living complexity of the subject itself. There were nights when words flowed like rivers, and others when silence stretched like deserts. Through it all, I held to the belief that science is not merely the accumulation of facts, but the weaving of meaning. And meaning, once shared, becomes the common inheritance of humankind.

To you, the reader: this book is both a map and a mirror. A map, to guide you through the terrain of biohybrid intelligence; and a mirror, to reflect the questions that science alone cannot answer. My hope is that as you turn these pages, you will not only gain knowledge but also feel the tremor of wonder — the sense that we stand, together, at the edge of something vast and unfinished. The horizon awaits, and it is my honor to invite you to sail toward it.

Mahdi Yousefian

Table of Contents

Chapter 1 – Foundations of Organoid Science

The Genesis of Stem Cell Research

The history of stem cell biology is the story of human curiosity confronting the deepest questions of identity and potential. Within the small boundaries of a Petri dish, scientists discovered cells that carried no fixed fate and yet the possibility of becoming nearly any cell type in the body.

By the late twentieth century, embryonic stem cells (ESCs) had been isolated from the inner cell mass of the blastocyst. These cells revealed the principle of pluripotency—the ability to differentiate into almost every tissue. They became a powerful model for understanding development and disease, yet their use raised profound ethical concerns, since their derivation required the destruction of early embryos.

The field transformed in 2006, when Shinya Yamanaka and his team in Japan demonstrated that adult fibroblast cells could be reprogrammed into a pluripotent state using only four transcription factors. These cells, called induced pluripotent stem cells (iPSCs), carried the same potential as ESCs but without the same ethical burden. With iPSCs, regenerative medicine became personal: patient-derived cells could be grown into neurons, muscle, or heart tissue, making "personalized biology" a reality.

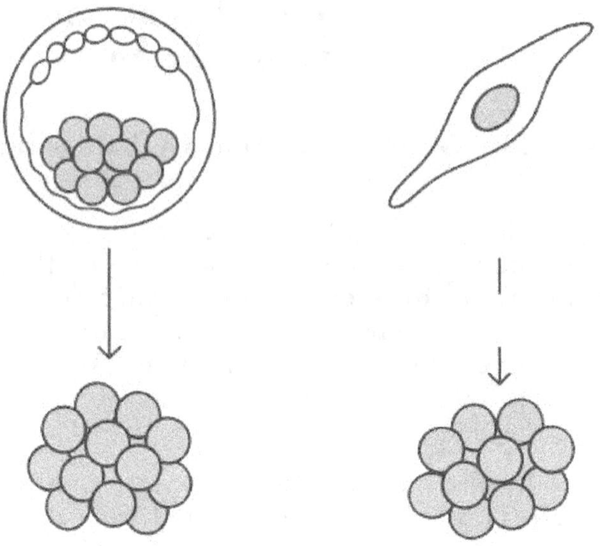

Figure1.1. Embryonic stem cells derived from the blastocyst compared with adult fibroblasts reprogrammed into iPSCs.

Table 1.1. Key comparison between ESCs and iPSCs

Feature	Embryonic Stem Cells (ESCs)	Induced Pluripotent Stem Cells (iPSCs)
Source	Inner cell mass of the blastocyst	Reprogrammed adult somatic cells (e.g., fibroblasts)
Pluripotency	Naturally pluripotent	Induced pluripotency via transcription factors (e.g., Oct4, Sox2, Klf4, c-Myc)
Ethical Concerns	High – requires destruction of human embryos	Lower – no embryos involved
Genetic Background	From donor embryo (not patient-specific)	Patient-specific, retains donor genome
Applications in Research	Gold standard for pluripotency, developmental biology	Disease modeling, regenerative medicine, personalized therapy
Limitations	Ethical issues, limited availability	Possible genetic/epigenetic abnormalities, variability

Pluripotency represents an extraordinary starting point, but its value lies in the ability to guide cells into specific fates. Among these, the neural lineage has become one of the most intensively studied.

The transition from pluripotency to neurons follows a carefully orchestrated sequence. First, stem cells are directed toward neural progenitors, which retain proliferative capacity but carry the molecular signature of the nervous system. These progenitors extend processes, establish polarity, and gradually commit to becoming neurons.

The process is not spontaneous—it requires precise cues. Growth factors, small molecules, and extracellular environments all contribute to instructing cells when to divide, when to pause, and when to specialize. Over time, these progenitors give rise to immature neurons, which extend dendrites and axons, forming the architecture of emerging networks.

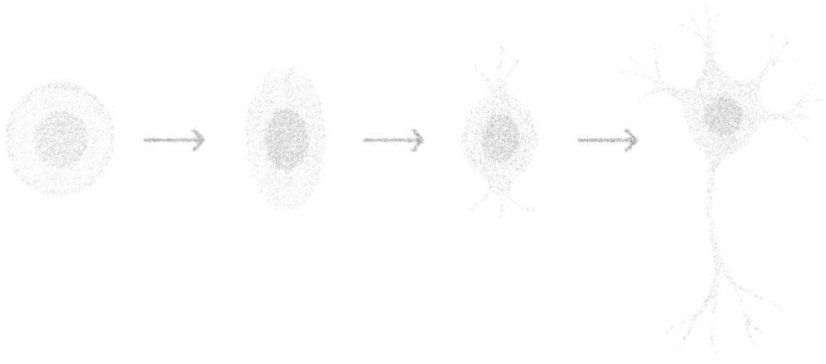

Figure1.2 Stages of neural differentiation: from pluripotent stem cell to neural progenitor to immature neuron to mature neuron.

1.3 Signaling Pathways and Molecular Guidance

The journey from stem cell to neuron is guided by an intricate choreography of molecular signals:

- BMP signaling normally promotes non-neural fates; its inhibition is essential for the initiation of neural identity.
- Wnt signaling establishes positional information, influencing whether progenitors adopt anterior or posterior neural fates.

- Notch signaling serves as a regulator of timing, maintaining the pool of progenitors until the moment is right for differentiation.

The balance of these pathways ensures both precision and diversity. It is through the interplay of these molecular "languages" that stem cells gradually construct networks that resemble, in miniature, the living brain.

Summary of Chapter 1

Stem cell research has transformed from an exploration of embryonic potential to a discipline capable of reprogramming adult cells and guiding them toward functional neurons. The field is more than a technical achievement: it is a story of transformation, ethics, and the enduring human ambition to recreate the building blocks of life. By mastering the dialogue of signals and pathways, scientists have begun to assemble systems that echo the complexity of the brain itself.

Chapter 2 – Building the Mini-Brain

Organoids are more than clusters of cells — they are architectures of memory, computation, and possibility. To build a "mini-brain" is not simply to grow tissue; it is to reenact, in vitro, the choreography of development that nature has refined across eons. In this chapter, we move from the raw potential of pluripotent stem cells to the emergent structures that echo cortical landscapes. We examine how scaffolds, timelines, and morphogenetic cues conspire to yield something that, under the microscope, resembles the beginnings of thought itself.

2.1 Biomimetic Scaffolds and Matrix Design

Every organoid begins with a microenvironment. Cells are not solitary agents; they are profoundly contextual, listening to the whispers of their neighbors and the mechanical signals of the substrate beneath them. To recreate this environment, scientists use biomimetic scaffolds — extracellular matrices (ECM) composed of proteins such as laminin and collagen, or synthetic hydrogels engineered to mimic their viscoelastic properties.

These matrices do more than hold cells together; they provide positional cues. A fibroblast feels rigidity differently from a neuron, and a progenitor cell interprets stiffness as a call to fate. Advances in 3D bioprinting now allow researchers to pattern these environments with extraordinary precision, arranging growth factors in gradients that mirror embryonic tissues. In this way, the scaffold is not just support — it is instruction.

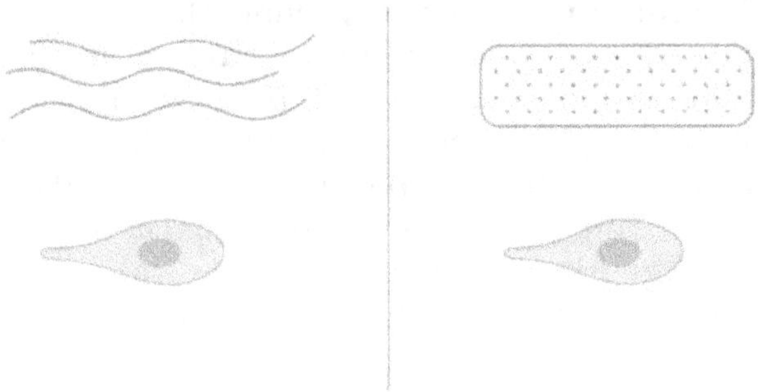

Figure2.1. Biomimetic scaffolds in organoid culture. Comparison of natural ECM proteins (laminin, collagen) with synthetic hydrogels, showing how they provide structural and biochemical cues for neural progenitor cells.

Table 2.1. Timeline of cerebral organoid development

Stage / Timepoint	Key Features	Notes
Day 0–7	Formation of embryoid bodies	Pluripotent cells aggregate and begin early polarity
Week 2–4	Emergence of neuroepithelial structures	Radial glia appear, early neural tube-like domains
Month 2–3	Cortical plate-like organization	Layered architecture, ventricular zone analogs
Month 4–6	Regionalization (forebrain-like, hippocampal-like areas)	Spontaneous activity detectable via MEA
Month 9–12	Mature neural networks with oscillatory activity	Still lacks vasculature; requires optimized culture

2.2 Timelines of Organoid Development

Organoid growth is a temporal narrative. In the first days, cells cluster, polarize, and form embryoid bodies — spherical precursors of higher organization. By the second week, these bodies begin to show germ-layer-like differentiation, producing neuroepithelial structures. Over the following months, cortical plates emerge, interspersed with rudimentary ventricle-like cavities.

A typical cerebral organoid may require two to six months to develop recognizable layered organization, with radial glia scaffolding neurons as they migrate outward. By one year, spontaneous network activity becomes detectable, resembling early developmental brain rhythms. Each stage is a recapitulation — compressed and imperfect — of human development itself.

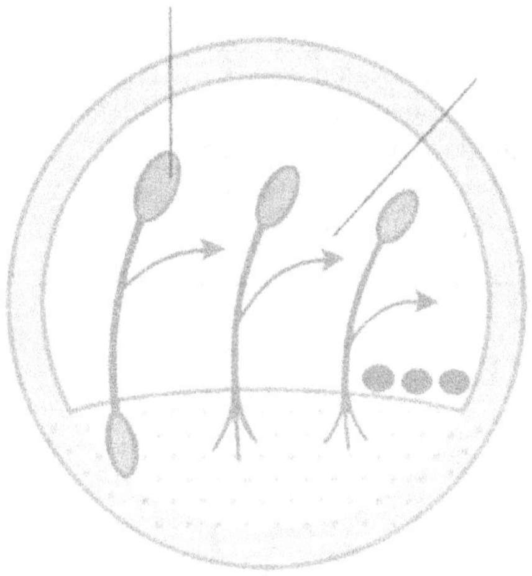

Figure 2.2. Morphogenesis of cortical layers in cerebral organoids. A schematic showing radial glia scaffolds, neuronal migration outward, and the emergence of rudimentary cortical zones.

2.3 Morphogenesis: Layers and Cortical Features

Morphogenesis is the silent architect of the mini-brain. Within the translucent tissue of an organoid, neural progenitors divide and align into structures evocative of the ventricular and subventricular zones. Over time, these progenitors give rise to neurons that migrate outward, forming rudimentary cortical layers.

Although organoids lack vasculature — a limitation that constrains their growth — they nonetheless exhibit hallmarks of regional specification: dorsal-ventral patterning, forebrain-like domains, and even the beginnings of hippocampal-like structures. Such emergent organization underscores the self-assembling nature of biology: given the right cues, cells seem to "remember" how to build a brain.

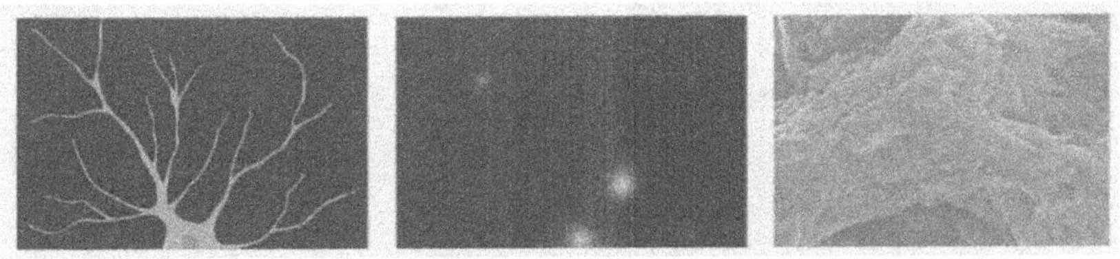

Figure 2.3. Imaging technologies applied to organoids.

Panel comparing confocal microscopy (neuronal networks), two-photon imaging (calcium sparks), and SEM (surface ultrastructure).

2.4 Imaging Frontiers: From Confocal to SEM

To witness the unfolding of these architectures, imaging technologies serve as windows into the miniature world. Confocal microscopy reveals networks of dendrites shimmering with fluorescent reporters, while two-photon imaging captures calcium sparks as neurons fire in synchrony. At the ultrastructural level, scanning electron microscopy (SEM) unveils landscapes of folded tissue, grooves, and synaptic contacts.

Increasingly, researchers couple imaging with computational analysis. Machine learning algorithms quantify neurite outgrowth, synapse density, and spatial organization, transforming pictures into data. In this convergence of biology and computation, the organoid ceases to be a mere specimen — it becomes a dataset, a living library of form and function.

Summary of Chapter 2

To build the mini-brain is to translate pluripotency into architecture. Through scaffolds that whisper mechanical truths, through developmental timelines that echo embryology, through morphogenetic choreography that yields cortical motifs, and through imaging that makes the invisible visible — organoids become more than experiments. They are laboratories of becoming, testaments to the fact that intelligence begins not in silicon, but in the patient unfolding of cells into form.

Chapter 3 – Culturing and Engineering Organoids

To culture an organoid is to negotiate with life itself. Unlike immortalized cell lines that bend easily to laboratory protocols, organoids demand patience, adaptation, and a constant recalibration of the environment in which they grow. In this chapter, we shift from theory to practice: how organoids are maintained, how they are engineered for robustness, and how the culture itself becomes a mirror of biological precision.

3.1 Static and Dynamic Cultivation

The earliest organoid cultures were grown in static conditions, where embryoid bodies floated in droplets of medium. Though simple, these systems faced severe diffusion limits. Nutrients and oxygen reached only the surface layers, while cells at the center starved, leading to necrosis.

Dynamic cultivation, by contrast, introduces constant mixing or rotation. Spinning bioreactors mimic the fluid dynamics of embryonic development, ensuring that every cell, deep within the organoid, encounters fresh nutrients and oxygen. This transition from static to dynamic systems was not merely technical — it was transformative, allowing organoids to expand in size and complexity beyond early limitations.

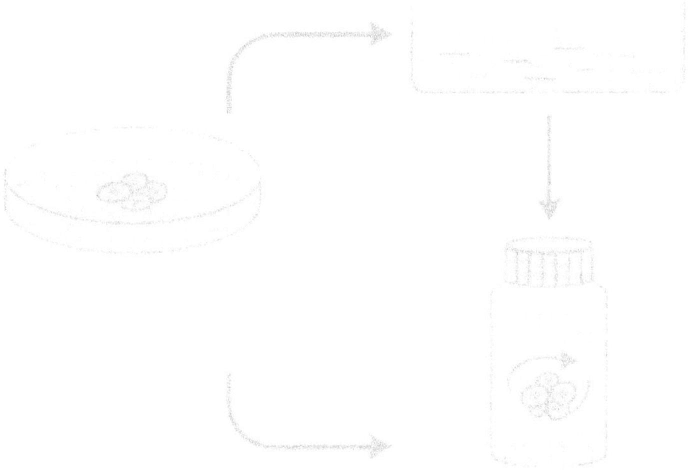

Figure 3.1. Culturing and engineering of organoids.

A schematic integrating static culture (droplet-based), dynamic spinning bioreactors, and medium optimization. The diagram shows how initial cell density, nutrient flow, and mechanical forces interact to influence growth, structural complexity, and reproducibility.

3.2 Bioreactors: Mechanics of Growth

Bioreactors represent the engineering heart of organoid science. In spinning or perfused systems, cells are suspended in a dance of turbulence and stability, exposed to gradients of oxygen and biochemical factors. The mechanical forces themselves influence growth: shear stress alters stem cell fate, while fluid motion enhances structural organization.

The design of bioreactors — from small-scale flasks to automated microfluidic systems — has made it possible to scale organoid production, bringing the dream of reproducible "mini-brains" closer to reality.

3.3 Cell Density and Medium Optimization

Organoid growth is exquisitely sensitive to the initial conditions. Too few cells, and the organoid fails to achieve structural integrity; too many, and overcrowding impairs differentiation. Researchers optimize not only density but also the recipe of the medium itself.

Growth factors such as EGF, FGF2, and BDNF provide proliferative signals, while small molecules like CHIR99021 tune Wnt signaling pathways. Serum-free formulations reduce variability, allowing results to be compared across laboratories. In the chemistry of the medium, one sees the convergence of biology and engineering: every molecule is a message, every concentration a decision.

3.4 Toward Standardization and Reproducibility

For organoid research to move from laboratory novelty to clinical application, reproducibility is paramount. Standardization efforts — from unified culture media to automated imaging protocols — aim to reduce variability across labs. Biobanks of well-characterized organoids are being developed, offering researchers "reference models" against which new experiments can be benchmarked.

Here, culture is more than maintenance: it is the scaffolding of a new scientific discipline, one that aspires to bring order to the creative chaos of biology.

Summary of Chapter 3

To culture organoids is to balance fragility and potential. From static droplets to dynamic bioreactors, from empirical recipes to standardized protocols, organoid cultivation represents a marriage of biology and engineering. It is in these controlled environments that stem cells learn to assemble into tissues that echo the brain — fragile yet profound, miniature yet infinite in implication.

Chapter 4 – Listening to the Living Circuit

If the organoid is a miniature brain, then its value lies not only in its structure but in its voice. Cells whisper to one another with electrical sparks and chemical pulses, weaving circuits that echo the earliest rhythms of cognition. To study organoids is not merely to watch them grow, but to learn how to listen — to translate the silent language of neurons into signals we can record, analyze, and perhaps one day understand.

4.1 Microelectrode Arrays (MEA)

Microelectrode arrays represent one of the most powerful tools for capturing organoid activity. By embedding electrodes beneath or around the tissue, scientists can detect extracellular field potentials — the bursts of activity generated when neurons fire in synchrony.

Unlike imaging, which offers snapshots of structure, MEAs reveal **real-time dynamics**: network oscillations, burst patterns, and even plastic changes as organoids respond to stimuli. The recordings resemble music without a score — a spontaneous composition of spikes that, with the right algorithms, can be mapped into coherent patterns.

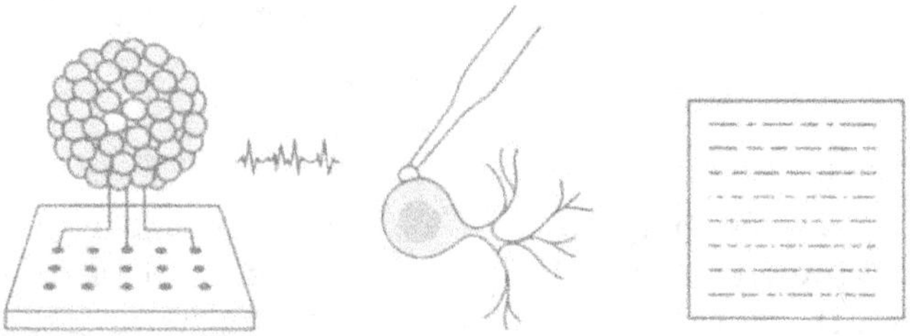

Figure 4.1 Recording techniques in organoid circuits.

A comparative schematic showing (left) MEA capturing network spikes across tissue, (middle) patch-clamp probing a single neuron, and (right) firing patterns displayed as raster plots.

Table 4.1. Comparison of recording methods in organoid studies

Method	Resolution Level	Strengths	Limitations
Microelectrode Arrays (MEA)	Network-level	Real-time activity, non-invasive, scalable	Limited spatial resolution
Patch-Clamp	Single-cell	High precision, ion-channel analysis	Technically demanding, low throughput
Calcium Imaging	Population of neurons	Visual dynamics, spatial mapping	Slower temporal resolution

4.2 Patch-Clamp and Electrophysiological Probing

For precision at the single-cell level, patch-clamp remains the gold standard. In this technique, a glass micropipette seals onto the membrane of a single neuron, allowing direct measurement of ion currents. With it, scientists can watch sodium and potassium channels open and close in response to voltage, capturing the elemental language of excitability.

Applied to organoids, patch-clamp studies show that these tissues are not passive clusters but active ensembles where individual neurons form functional synapses. Through such methods, we glimpse the microcosm of connectivity that underlies cognition.

4.3 Neural Firing Patterns and Synaptic Plasticity

Electrical activity is not random — it carries meaning in its rhythms. In organoids, spontaneous firing emerges over weeks, evolving from disorganized bursts into patterns resembling early developmental brain waves. These signals reveal both the promise and the limitation of organoid models: they are not fully brains, but they carry echoes of developmental logic.

Synaptic plasticity — the ability of connections to strengthen or weaken — has also been observed. With repeated stimulation, organoids exhibit potentiation, a hallmark of learning at the cellular level. To observe this is to witness the dawn of memory in tissue that has never seen a world.

Summary of Chapter 4

To listen to organoids is to cross a threshold. From the silence of static tissue emerges a symphony of spikes, bursts, and rhythms that testify to the living circuitry within. Through MEAs, patch-clamp, and imaging, scientists do more than measure — they interpret. In the language of voltage and current, organoids tell us that they are not inert: they are active, plastic, and perhaps, in their own miniature way, already thinking.

Chapter 5 – Multimodal Stimulation and Recording

Organoids are not passive clusters of cells. They perceive, respond, and adapt to the cues in their environment. To understand these miniature brains, scientists must move beyond passive recording and engage in a true dialogue: stimulation and response. In this chapter, we explore the emerging toolbox of multimodal stimulation and recording — from beams of light that trigger neurons to acoustic waves that ripple through tissues, from microfluidic forces that stretch cells to calcium signals that illuminate networks. Together, these methods form a symphony of inputs and outputs, revealing the plasticity and complexity of organoid circuits.

5.1 Optogenetic Modulation

Optogenetics provides unparalleled precision. By introducing light-sensitive ion channels (such as **Channelrhodopsin-2**), neurons can be activated with millisecond accuracy. This technique transforms organoids into systems where causality can be tested: a pulse of blue light in one region evokes a wave of activity in another.

- **Strengths**: High temporal precision, targeted activation.
- **Limitations**: Requires genetic modification, light penetration limited in dense tissues.

Table 5.1. Multimodal stimulation and recording approaches in organoid research

Method	Mode of Stimulation/Recording	Key Applications	Limitations
Optogenetics	Light-based activation via opsins	Millisecond control of neuronal firing, causal mapping	Requires genetic modification, light penetration limited
Mechanical stimulation	Microfluidic flow, stretch, or pressure	Modeling development, mechanosensitivity, growth	Less precise, risk of tissue damage
Acoustic stimulation	Ultrasound, sound waves	Non-invasive deep modulation, network studies	Lower spatial specificity, possible heating
Calcium Imaging	Fluorescence from Ca^{2+} indicators	Mapping functional connectivity, network activity	Slow temporal resolution, indirect measure
Electrophysiology (MEA)	Electrical recording of spikes/bursts	Real-time network activity, high temporal precision	Limited spatial resolution
Multimodal integration	Combining multiple methods	Comprehensive view of organoid circuits, cross-validation	Complex analysis, high data processing demands

5.2 Mechanical and Acoustic Stimulation

Organoids are also sensitive to forces. Microfluidic platforms apply shear stress, stretch, or pressure, mimicking the physical microenvironment of development. These methods are invaluable for studying how neurons and glia respond to biomechanical cues.

Acoustic stimulation, using ultrasound or patterned sound waves, provides a non-invasive way to modulate activity deep within the tissue. Low-intensity ultrasound has been shown to enhance neuronal firing and even induce plasticity in organoids.

- Strengths: Non-invasive, scalable.
- Limitations: Lower spatial resolution; risk of overstimulation or mechanical stress.

5.4 Synchronizing Data Across Modalities

The future lies in integration. No single method captures the entirety of organoid activity. By combining electrophysiology (for timing), calcium imaging (for spatial patterns), and optogenetics (for causal perturbation), researchers can generate multimodal datasets that approach a holistic view of living circuits.

This integration is computationally demanding. Advanced algorithms, from deep learning models to Bayesian frameworks, are being developed to merge heterogeneous data streams into coherent representations of organoid function.

Summary of Chapter 5

To stimulate and record from organoids is to invite them into conversation. Light can make them speak, pressure can shape their growth, sound can stir their rhythms, and calcium flashes reveal their hidden choreography. When integrated, these methods allow us to move from fragments of signal to symphonies of activity — a step closer to understanding whether these organoids are not only alive, but intelligent.

Chapter 6 – Editing the Blueprint: CRISPR-Cas9

If organoids are living testaments to self-organization, then CRISPR is the sculptor's chisel — a tool to rewrite the very language of life. With it, scientists do not merely observe organoids; they design them, engineering disease models, correcting genetic errors, and even enhancing biological performance. To edit DNA is to reach into the instruction manual of nature and alter the rules by which cells build themselves. It is both an act of precision and of audacity.

6.1 Designing gRNA: Precision Tools

At the heart of CRISPR-Cas9 lies the guide RNA (gRNA), a short sequence that directs the Cas9 nuclease to its target in the genome. Designing this gRNA is a process of exquisite specificity: too short, and it risks binding unintended sites; too permissive, and off-target edits can destabilize the entire experiment.

Modern algorithms scan the genome for target motifs, ranking candidates by predicted efficiency and specificity. Once chosen, the gRNA becomes a molecular compass, bringing Cas9 directly to the locus of interest. The act resembles navigation in a vast library: the genome as millions of volumes, and CRISPR as the bookmark that finds the single line to be changed.

6.2 Disease Models: Alzheimer's and ALS

One of the most transformative uses of CRISPR in organoids has been the modeling of neurodegenerative diseases.

In Alzheimer's disease, specific mutations in genes such as APP, PSEN1, and APOE4 are introduced into stem cells before organoid differentiation. As these cells form cerebral organoids, they begin to exhibit hallmark pathologies: amyloid plaques, tau tangles, and network dysfunction. Unlike mouse models, which only approximate the human condition, these organoids carry human mutations in human tissue, bringing researchers closer to the biological truth.

In amyotrophic lateral sclerosis (ALS), mutations in SOD1 or C9orf72 have been engineered into organoids to study motor neuron degeneration. Researchers watch as motor neurons lose their connectivity, glial cells adopt toxic phenotypes, and the organoid becomes a living microcosm of disease. Here, CRISPR is not only a modeling tool — it is a time machine, compressing years of pathology into weeks of laboratory growth.

6.3 Enhancing Neuronal Performance

CRISPR is not limited to simulating disease. Increasingly, it is being used to enhance function. By editing regulatory genes that govern synaptic proteins, scientists have produced organoids with stronger or more reliable neuronal firing. Manipulating ion channel genes has yielded cells with altered excitability, while modification of synaptic vesicle proteins has changed the efficiency of neurotransmitter release.

Such work raises profound questions: if organoids can be engineered for performance, do we risk creating tissue that surpasses natural biology? At what point does enhancement move from science into speculation about "designed intelligence"? The ethical debates remain unsettled, but the science advances nonetheless.

6.4 Molecular Readouts: PCR and NGS

Editing is only half the story. Verification is essential. Once CRISPR has been deployed, researchers must confirm whether the intended changes occurred and whether unintended edits slipped through.

Polymerase Chain Reaction (PCR) provides the first layer of verification, amplifying the target sequence to check for modifications. For finer resolution, Next-Generation Sequencing (NGS) offers a genome-wide perspective, identifying both on-target and off-target edits.

These molecular readouts transform CRISPR from a black box into a transparent process. Without them, the promise of precision would remain unfulfilled, as every edit must be proven before it can be trusted.

Ethical Dimensions of Genome Editing in Organoids

Behind every technical triumph lies a philosophical shadow. When scientists alter DNA in organoids, they are reshaping tissues that may one day exhibit features of cognition. Is it permissible to engineer disease into such tissues, knowing that they may develop signatures of suffering? Is enhancement an act of progress, or of hubris?

Global frameworks remain cautious. Most guidelines, from the ISSCR (International Society for Stem Cell Research) to regional bioethics committees, permit genome editing in organoids but demand strict oversight. The line is clear: organoids must not cross into territory where sentience or consciousness is plausible. Yet as CRISPR technology becomes more sophisticated, that boundary grows harder to police.

Summary of Chapter 6

CRISPR-Cas9 has revolutionized organoid science, giving researchers the power not only to observe biology but to engineer it. Through gRNA design, disease modeling, neuronal enhancement, and molecular readouts, scientists now sculpt the organoid genome with extraordinary precision. Yet with this power comes responsibility: to wield CRISPR is to carry both the scalpel of healing and the sword of ethical dilemma. In the miniature circuits of organoids, the future of biology is being drafted — one nucleotide at a time.

Chapter 7 – Profiling the Organoid

If cultivation and engineering give organoids their form, then profiling gives them their story. To profile is to measure, decode, and classify the countless molecules that sustain life — from transcripts that hum in the nucleus to proteins folded into intricate machines. In organoid science, profiling transforms tissue from a black box into a map of activity. It allows us to see not just what organoids look like, but who they are, what they are becoming, and how they differ across individuals and conditions.

Unlike classical histology, which provided snapshots of tissue, modern profiling is multidimensional. Genomics, transcriptomics, proteomics, and metabolomics now converge to create a comprehensive atlas of organoid biology. This chapter explores the technologies, challenges, and implications of profiling organoids, focusing on RNA sequencing, single-cell approaches, proteomics, and the integration of large-scale datasets.

7.1 RNA-Seq and Single-Cell Transcriptomics

The genome is stable, but the transcriptome is alive. Every cell within an organoid activates different sets of genes depending on its state, its environment, and its destiny. RNA sequencing (RNA-Seq) provides a global overview of this dynamic landscape, capturing which genes are being expressed and at what levels.

Single-cell RNA-Seq takes this one step further. Instead of averaging across thousands of cells, it dissects the individuality of each cell. In a cerebral organoid, one cell might reveal itself as a radial glial progenitor, while its neighbor expresses markers of immature neurons. This single-cell resolution has revealed surprising diversity: even in "simple" organoids, dozens of distinct cell states coexist, interacting in patterns that echo human cortical development.

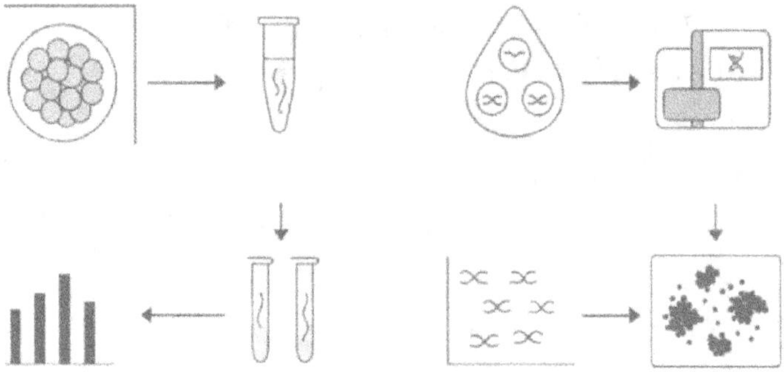

Figure 7.1. RNA-Seq and single-cell transcriptomics in organoids.Schematic showing bulk RNA-Seq workflow (tissue → mRNA isolation → sequencing) compared with single-cell RNA-Seq (individual cells sorted → transcriptome profiled → clustering of cell types

7.2 Mapping the Proteome

Transcripts tell us what cells intend to do, but proteins reveal what they actually do. Proteomics uses mass spectrometry and antibody-based assays to catalog the proteins within an organoid. Beyond quantity, proteomics uncovers post-translational modifications — phosphorylation, ubiquitination, glycosylation — that control protein activity.

In brain organoids, proteomic profiling has revealed the emergence of synaptic machinery long before it is visible under a microscope. Proteins such as synapsin, PSD-95, and NMDA receptors are detected, showing that cells are not only differentiating but wiring themselves into functional circuits.

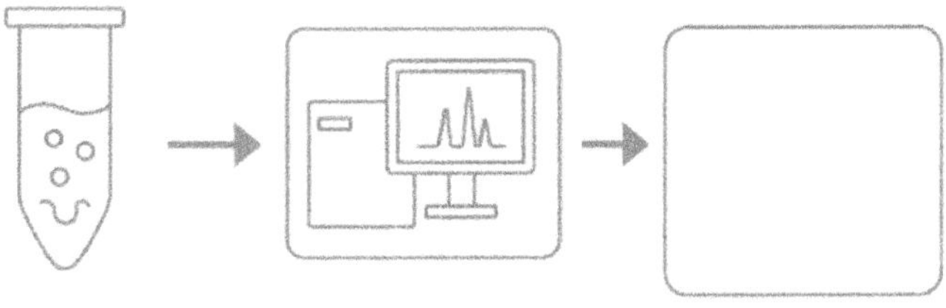

Figure 7.2. Proteomic profiling of organoids.

Workflow illustration of protein extraction → mass spectrometry analysis → identification of synaptic and signaling proteins in organoid development.

7.3 Omics Data Quality and Databases

With great data comes great responsibility. RNA-Seq and proteomics generate vast datasets, but their value depends on quality control and standardization. Batch effects, sequencing errors, and sample variability can distort results. For this reason, organoid researchers rely on pipelines that filter noise, normalize data, and benchmark against known standards.

The global scientific community has also begun building shared databases of organoid profiles. These repositories function as atlases: researchers can compare their data against public datasets, validate results, and even predict new biological patterns. AI-driven tools increasingly mine these databases, identifying hidden correlations across thousands of experiments.

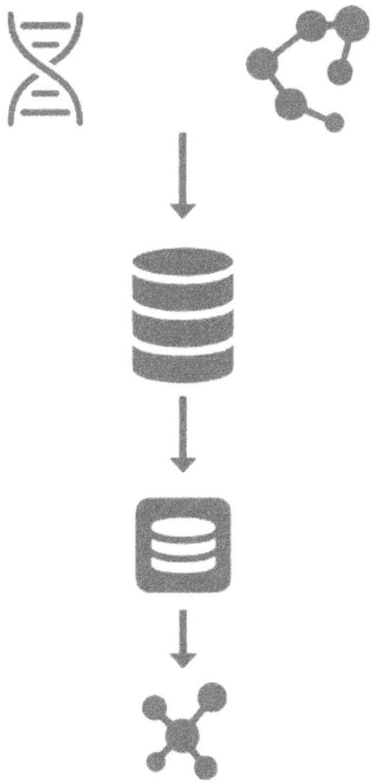

Figure 7.3. Omics integration in organoid research.

A diagram showing the convergence of transcriptomics, proteomics, and metabolomics into shared databases, analyzed by AI pipelines for systems-level insights.

The Future of Organoid Profiling

The next frontier is not only to profile but to predict. By combining multi-omics with machine learning, researchers aim to forecast how organoids will respond to drugs, mutations, or environmental cues. Imagine a future where a patient's own cells are grown into an organoid, profiled in real time, and used to simulate decades of biology within weeks.

Such ambitions raise profound questions: if profiling can capture the essence of individuality, are organoids mere models, or are they partial representations of the self? And if data is the new genome, how should society regulate its use? Privacy, consent, and ownership of biological data become as urgent as the science itself.

Summary of Chapter 7

Profiling organoids is the act of listening not to their spikes or waves, but to their molecules. RNA-Seq and single-cell methods reveal transcriptional diversity, proteomics uncovers the machinery of function, and omics databases weave individual experiments into a global map. As data grows, so too does our responsibility to interpret, regulate, and safeguard it. In the atlas of organoid profiling, science moves closer to seeing not only the biology of these tissues but their potential to mirror the human condition.

Chapter 8 – Artificial Intelligence Meets Biology

The story of organoids is not only biological; it is computational. As organoids grow in complexity, they generate signals — electrical, molecular, morphological — that surpass the ability of human intuition to interpret. To make sense of these vast datasets, researchers increasingly turn to artificial intelligence (AI), forging a new symbiosis between living tissue and silicon algorithms.

AI in organoid research does more than analyze; it predicts, classifies, and even suggests interventions. From electrophysiological spikes to high-resolution imaging datasets, machine learning transforms raw data into insights. This chapter explores the major intersections of AI and organoid science: from signal classification to predictive modeling, from neural networks to hybrid architectures that merge organic and artificial computation.

8.1 Signal Classification: SVM and Random Forest

Organoid circuits recorded by microelectrode arrays (MEAs) or patch-clamp generate thousands of electrical spikes every second. Distinguishing noise from meaningful patterns requires advanced classifiers.

- Support Vector Machines (SVMs): Particularly effective in separating nonlinear clusters of firing patterns. They excel in detecting abnormal rhythms, such as epileptiform activity in cortical organoids.

- Random Forests: Useful for multi-dimensional datasets, combining numerous decision trees to identify which features (frequency, burst duration, amplitude) best distinguish one condition from another.

In early studies, these classifiers have differentiated between healthy and disease-model organoids, providing a diagnostic lens at cellular resolution.

Table 8.1. Applications of AI in organoid research

AI Method	Data Type	Application in Organoids	Strengths	Limitations
Support Vector Machines	Electrophysiology (MEA)	Classifying spike patterns, detecting abnormal rhythms	High accuracy in small datasets	Sensitive to parameter tuning
Random Forests	Multimodal signals	Feature ranking, disease vs. healthy classification	Handles large feature sets well	Less interpretable
Convolutional Neural Nets	Imaging data	Identifying structural motifs, cortical layers	Strong in spatial recognition	Requires large labeled datasets
Recurrent Neural Nets (LSTM)	Time-series (calcium waves, spikes)	Predicting dynamics, oscillations	Captures long-term dependencies	Training-intensive
Reinforcement Learning	Closed-loop interaction	Stimulus-response experiments, adaptive control	Enables bi-directional training	Still experimental, low reproducibility

8.2 CNNs for Imaging, RNNs for Dynamics

Where electrophysiology captures temporal events, imaging provides spatial maps. Organoids imaged with confocal microscopy, calcium imaging, or fMRI-like approaches produce terabytes of visual data.

Convolutional Neural Networks (CNNs): Excel at identifying structural motifs — cortical folds, ventricular zones, or abnormal morphologies. In brain tumor organoids, CNNs have been used to detect growth patterns predictive of malignancy.

Recurrent Neural Networks (RNNs) and Long Short-Term Memory (LSTM) models: Handle time-series data. Applied to firing patterns or calcium waves, they predict how activity evolves, detecting hidden rhythms invisible to classical analysis.

Together, CNNs and RNNs provide a two-eyed view: one captures form, the other captures flow.

Table 8.2. Comparative advantages of AI vs. traditional analysis

Dimension	Traditional Analysis	AI-Based Analysis
Scalability	Limited to small datasets	Handles terabytes of omics and imaging data
Pattern Detection	Pre-defined statistical measures	Learns hidden, nonlinear patterns
Interpretability	Transparent but less flexible	High accuracy but often black-box
Speed	Manual, time-consuming	Automated, real-time or near real-time
Predictive Capacity	Correlation-based, limited foresight	Strong forecasting of drug/genetic outcomes
Integration of Modalities	Rare, labor-intensive	Easily combines electrophysiology, imaging, omics

8.3 Predictive Modeling of Neural Behavior

Beyond classification lies prediction. Using deep learning, researchers now train models to anticipate how organoids will respond to stimulation, drugs, or genetic edits.

For example:

- Organoids treated with antiepileptic compounds can be modeled to predict whether spiking activity will normalize.
- Genetic modifications introduced with CRISPR are simulated computationally to forecast whether they will enhance or impair network connectivity.
- In some pioneering studies, reinforcement learning frameworks have been used to train AI to "communicate" with organoids, sending input stimuli and receiving responses in closed-loop experiments.

This predictive capacity transforms organoids into living laboratories of future biology. Instead of trial and error, AI-guided models accelerate discovery, saving time and resources.

8.4 The Architecture of Biohybrid Intelligence

Perhaps the most provocative idea is that organoids and AI are not merely tools for one another but potential partners. Hybrid systems are emerging where biological activity provides data for artificial networks, and in turn, artificial networks suggest stimuli for the organoid.

This closed-loop cycle blurs the line between simulation and embodiment. Is the organoid teaching the AI, or is the AI training the organoid? In these systems, information flows in both directions, producing a form of computation that neither biology nor silicon could achieve alone.

8.5 Challenges and Ethical Reflections

With power comes responsibility. AI-driven profiling of organoids risks overinterpretation — seeing intelligence where only noise exists. Ethical questions also arise:

- If AI algorithms confirm that organoids exhibit learning-like behavior, should these tissues be afforded new moral consideration?

- Who owns the datasets generated by patient-derived organoids, and how should they be used in AI training pipelines?

- Could AI itself be biased in its interpretation of organoid signals, perpetuating errors in diagnosis or therapy?

These concerns remind us that AI is not neutral; it is shaped by its design and its datasets. To merge AI with organoids is not only a scientific act but also a cultural and ethical one.

Summary of Chapter 8

Artificial intelligence has become both microscope and telescope for organoid research: a microscope, revealing hidden details in datasets too vast for the eye; a telescope, predicting futures that biology alone cannot foresee. From SVMs and random forests to deep neural networks, AI transforms organoids from passive tissues into interactive systems of biohybrid intelligence. Yet as algorithms grow more powerful, ethical vigilance must keep pace, ensuring that the union of biology and computation remains a tool for knowledge, not exploitation.

Chapter 9 – Toward Biohybrid Intelligence

The term *biohybrid intelligence* captures a vision that is both radical and inevitable: that the boundaries between living tissue and artificial computation are not fixed, but porous. If organoids can sense, learn, and adapt, and if artificial intelligence can process, model, and predict, then the union of the two may open a new era of cognition — neither entirely biological, nor entirely machine, but something in between.

In this chapter, we move beyond organoid profiling and AI analysis to ask: what does it mean to couple these systems in real time? What architectures allow such integration? How can signals be exchanged across the biological–digital divide? And, most provocatively, how should the performance of such hybrid systems be measured?

9.1 Architectures of Organoid–Silicon Integration

Integration begins with interfaces. On one side, organoids communicate through spikes, calcium waves, and molecular signaling. On the other, silicon circuits speak in voltage, code, and algorithms. The bridge is built through bioelectronic devices such as microelectrode arrays, optogenetic light delivery systems, and microfluidic actuators.

microelectrode arrays, optogenetic light delivery systems, and microfluidic actuators.

Several architectures are being tested:

- Unidirectional systems: where organoids act as sensors and AI interprets their outputs. For example, organoid responses to toxins can be translated into computational alerts.

- Bidirectional systems: where AI not only reads but also writes, stimulating organoids with light or current while analyzing their responses. This closed-loop interaction resembles dialogue rather than observation.

- Embedded systems: where organoids are placed directly within computational hardware, serving as living processors whose plasticity augments the fixed logic of silicon.

Each architecture represents a different philosophy: organoids as data sources, as partners, or as processors in their own right.

9.2 Data Exchange: From Spikes to Code

At the heart of biohybrid intelligence lies the problem of translation. Neural spikes must be transformed into machine-readable code, while AI outputs must be rendered into biological stimuli. This exchange is far from trivial.

- Encoding biological signals: Spike trains are digitized, compressed, and classified, then mapped onto symbolic or numerical representations.
- Decoding AI commands: Computational instructions are converted into optical or electrical stimuli — a pulse of blue light, a timed current — that the organoid can interpret.
- Synchronization: Advanced clocking systems ensure that biological time (slower, noisy, variable) and digital time (fast, precise) can align just enough to permit coherent interaction.

These exchanges are not perfect translations, but they are sufficient to allow a rudimentary form of communication — a "lingua franca" of hybrid systems.

9.3 Evaluating Biohybrid Performance

The challenge is not only to build biohybrids but to measure their performance. Traditional metrics of AI — accuracy, efficiency, throughput — do not capture the plastic, evolving nature of organoids. Conversely, biological measures like synaptic plasticity or metabolic activity may not reflect computational utility.

Emerging criteria include:

- Adaptability: Does the hybrid system improve its performance over time when exposed to new tasks?
- Robustness: How stable is the integration when faced with noise, variability, or perturbation?
- Novelty generation: Can the system produce solutions or behaviors not explicitly programmed or trained?
- Energy efficiency: Since neurons consume far less power than silicon, can biohybrids leverage this advantage?

In some pilot experiments, organoid–AI hybrids have learned simple tasks such as pattern recognition more flexibly than silicon alone. Though primitive, these results hint at a future where evaluation itself may require new philosophical frameworks: What counts as intelligence? What counts as agency?

The Philosophical Horizon

To speak of biohybrid intelligence is to confront questions larger than science. If such systems exhibit learning, memory, and adaptation, are they mere tools, or do they deserve recognition as novel entities? Do they belong to the realm of machines, or should they be considered as living collaborators?

Some argue that the value lies not in whether biohybrids are "conscious," but in their ability to **expand human cognition**. Just as telescopes extended our vision and calculators extended our arithmetic, biohybrids may extend our capacity to perceive and reason. Others, however, warn of anthropomorphism — the temptation to see intelligence where there is only sophisticated noise.

What is certain is that biohybrid intelligence is not science fiction. It is being built, cell by cell and algorithm by algorithm, in laboratories around the world.

Summary of Chapter 9

Biohybrid intelligence is the next frontier: the merging of living organoids with artificial systems to create platforms that learn, adapt, and perhaps even innovate. Through architectures of integration, translation of signals, and novel performance metrics, these systems challenge our definitions of both biology and computation. As science advances, philosophy must keep pace, for in biohybrids we may glimpse the first outlines of a new kind of mind — neither wholly human nor wholly machine, but something profoundly new.

Chapter 10 – Ethics and Global Frameworks

Organoids stand at the threshold of possibility and responsibility. To culture a cerebral organoid, to stimulate it, and to edit its genome are not only technical acts but moral choices. Ethics in organoid science is not an afterthought; it is the scaffolding that determines how far and how safely the field can advance. As these living models come closer to mimicking the complexity of the human brain, society faces new dilemmas: What constitutes consciousness? Where must society draw its boundaries? Who decides what is permissible?

This chapter explores these questions, situating organoid research within a global framework of ethical, cultural, and regulatory considerations.

10.1 Defining Consciousness: Science or Philosophy?

Perhaps the most pressing ethical question is whether organoids could one day achieve a form of consciousness. Scientists argue that organoids lack the structural and systemic integration of a full brain — no sensory inputs, no body, no long-range circuits. Yet organoids already display network oscillations reminiscent of fetal brain activity.

Philosophers remind us that consciousness is not simply a product of complexity but a qualitative phenomenon — the *what it is like* to have experience. At present, there is no evidence that organoids are conscious, but the possibility alone shifts the debate. Should ethical frameworks anticipate consciousness, even if it is uncertain?

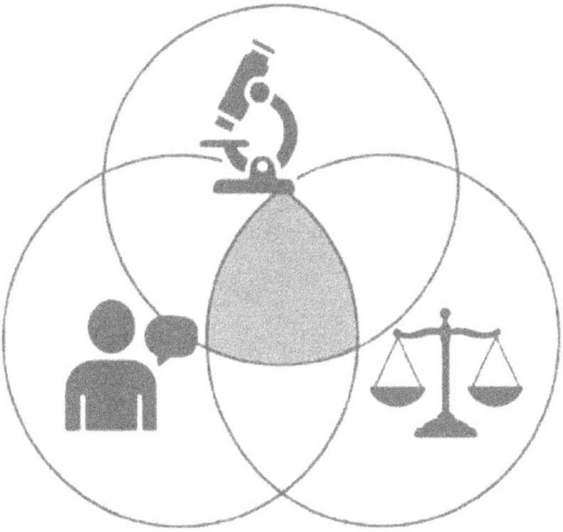

Figure 10.1. Ethical dimensions of organoid research

(A schematic diagram showing three intersecting domains: Scientific Progress, Ethical Boundaries, and Societal Perception. The overlap represents "Responsible Innovation.")

Table 10.1. Ethical and regulatory perspectives on organoid research

Framework / Region	Key Ethical Focus	Strengths	Limitations
FDA (USA)	Clinical safety, patient protection	Strong focus on therapeutic translation	Limited engagement with philosophical issues
EMA (Europe)	Harmonization, patient rights	Emphasizes cross-border consistency	Slower approval process
ISSCR (Global)	Broad ethical guidance, research limits	Sets international standards, flexible updates	Non-binding; relies on voluntary compliance
Public Opinion	Societal trust, cultural acceptance	Encourages dialogue, reflects diverse values	Easily swayed by misinformation

10.2 Societal and Cultural Reflections

Ethical concerns are not confined to the laboratory. Different cultures interpret organoid research through their own philosophical and religious lenses:

- In some traditions, the brain is seen as the seat of the soul, raising deep concern about creating brain-like tissue in vitro.
- Others celebrate organoid research as an extension of medicine, offering new hope for treating neurodegenerative diseases.
- Public perception also matters: media portrayals of "mini-brains" often exaggerate capabilities, fueling both excitement and fear.

Without careful communication, mistrust can slow research or lead to premature bans. Building public dialogue is therefore as essential as scientific rigor.

10.3 Guidelines: FDA, EMA, ISSCR

To balance innovation with responsibility, regulatory bodies have issued frameworks:

- FDA (United States): Focuses on translational aspects — ensuring organoid-derived therapies are safe for clinical trials.

- EMA (European Medicines Agency): Emphasizes cross-border ethical harmonization, particularly for regenerative medicine.

- ISSCR (International Society for Stem Cell Research): Provides global ethical guidelines, including restrictions on experiments that might induce advanced neural features.

These guidelines stress transparency, oversight, and limitation. Researchers must report methods, justify endpoints, and avoid experiments that risk creating sentient-like organoids. Yet enforcement remains uneven, leaving gaps in accountability.

Summary of Chapter 10

Ethics and governance are not external to organoid science; they are woven into its very future. Consciousness debates force us to redefine thresholds, cultural reflections remind us that science is never value-free, and guidelines from FDA, EMA, and ISSCR attempt to balance promise with precaution. The path forward requires dialogue among scientists, ethicists, policymakers, and the public. Only by embedding responsibility into discovery can organoids serve not only as models of biology but as models of how science itself should evolve.

Chapter 11 – Future Horizons

The story of organoids is still unfinished. What we see today in the laboratory — clusters of cells, electrical bursts, molecular signatures — may one day evolve into platforms that transform medicine, intelligence, and even our self-understanding. To write about the future is always to risk imagination outpacing reality, yet in organoid science, the horizon is closer than we think.

This chapter outlines possible futures: near-term innovations (5 years), mid-term transformations (10 years), and long-term revolutions (30 years and beyond). It considers applications in precision medicine, artificial intelligence, and the emerging bio-economy. The aim is not prediction, but preparation: to think about the directions in which science might grow, and the choices humanity will face along the way.

11.1 Roadmap: 5, 10, 30 Years

- **5 Years**: Standardization of organoid culture, improved reproducibility, and integration of organoid databases into personalized medicine. Small-scale clinical applications begin, particularly in drug screening.

- **10 Years**: Organoids incorporated into hybrid AI platforms. Ethical frameworks mature; regulatory agencies create clearer policies. Organoids begin to serve as predictive avatars for individual patients.
- **30 Years**: Emergence of biohybrid systems as part of mainstream computing and medicine. Potentially, organoids contribute to novel architectures of cognition — systems that extend human intelligence itself.

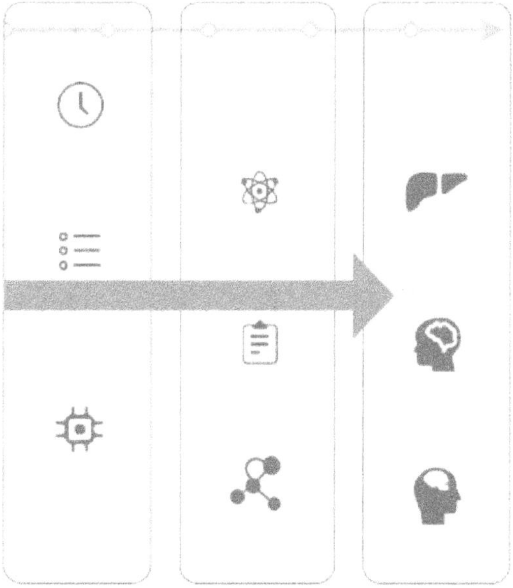

Figure 11.1. Timeline of organoid science.

A schematic roadmap showing projected advances at 5, 10, and 30 years.

Table 11.1. Future scenarios for organoid research

Time Horizon	Key Developments	Potential Impact	Challenges
5 Years	Standardization, organoid biobanks, drug screening	Faster clinical translation	Reproducibility, early ethical concerns
10 Years	Patient-specific avatars, AI integration	Personalized medicine, hybrid intelligence	Regulatory frameworks, data security
30 Years	Biohybrid cognition, bio-economy expansion	New industries, extended human intelligence	Societal acceptance, deep ethical dilemmas

11.2 Organoids in Precision Medicine and AI

One of the most promising applications lies in precision medicine. By deriving organoids directly from patients, doctors can test therapies in vitro before applying them in vivo. Instead of a generic treatment plan, medicine becomes individualized: a drug is not prescribed because it works on average, but because it works on your cells.

At the same time, organoids will increasingly merge with artificial intelligence. AI will analyze omics profiles, electrical recordings, and imaging data, creating digital twins of organoids that allow simulation and prediction. In some cases, AI may even learn directly from organoid activity, creating a feedback loop between biology and computation.

11.3 Organoids and the Bio-Economy

Beyond science and medicine, organoids may reshape the global economy. A "bio-economy" driven by living systems could emerge, with organoids used for drug discovery, toxicity testing, neurological modeling, and hybrid computation. Investment will follow, creating new industries at the intersection of biotechnology and information technology.

This expansion will not be without risks: inequality of access, intellectual property battles, and ethical debates about ownership of living data. Yet the potential benefits — cures for neurodegenerative diseases, sustainable bio-computing, and new industries — are vast.

Summary of Chapter 11

The horizon of organoid science is not a distant line but a moving frontier. In five years, reproducibility will redefine credibility; in ten years, organoid avatars will enter the clinic; in thirty years, biohybrid intelligence may reshape human thought. Alongside these advances, a bio-economy will rise, raising questions about equity, ethics, and access. To imagine the future is to recognize that the story of organoids is not only about biology but about humanity itself — its hopes, fears, and choices in the face of possibility.

12.1 Returning to the Beginning

Every scientific journey eventually circles back to its origins. In the story of organoid intelligence, the return to the beginning is not merely symbolic—it is essential. To look ahead, we must re-examine where we began: a single cell, undifferentiated, holding within it the vast potential of all that life could become. The past eleven chapters have traced this remarkable trajectory, from the discovery of stem cells to the engineering of biohybrid systems that whisper of cognition. But in order to envision the future, we must anchor ourselves once again in that first moment of discovery, when biology and imagination collided.

Science has always been a cycle of forgetting and remembering. Each paradigm shift forces us to abandon certain assumptions, only to rediscover them later under a new light. Organoid intelligence embodies this cycle. The idea that a cluster of cells in a dish could reveal truths about human thought would have seemed implausible just a generation ago. Yet here we stand, on the threshold of a new era, and the question emerges: how did we arrive here, and what does our origin tell us about where we are heading?

Revisiting Stem Cell Genesis

The dawn of organoid research can be traced to the late twentieth century, when embryonic stem cells were first isolated from the inner cell mass of the blastocyst. These cells, with their property of pluripotency, were hailed as a biological tabula rasa. Scientists marveled at their potential to differentiate into nearly any tissue. Yet, the ethical burden was heavy: deriving embryonic stem cells required the destruction of human embryos. It was a discovery both celebrated and contested, lighting the spark for decades of scientific and philosophical debate.

Fast forward to 2006, when Shinya Yamanaka's work on induced pluripotent stem cells (iPSCs) changed the landscape. By introducing just four transcription factors, ordinary fibroblast cells were reprogrammed back into a pluripotent state. For the first time, humanity possessed a renewable, ethically sustainable source of stem cells. The door to personalized biology swung open: a patient's own cells could be harvested, reprogrammed, and used to model disease or test therapies. This was more than technical progress; it was a philosophical shift. Life could be reset.

This genesis remains central to the story of organoid intelligence. Without pluripotency—without the capacity to return to the beginning—there could be no organoids, no living neural circuits, and no hybrid systems of biology and computation.

Organoids: Microcosms of Development

The subsequent chapters in this book detailed how pluripotent stem cells were guided into complex three-dimensional structures. Organoids, these miniature self-organizing tissues, are not mere clusters of cells; they are developmental processes captured in microcosm. To watch an organoid form is to witness biology replaying its ancient script, condensed and accelerated.

But the return to the beginning is not only technical—it is metaphorical. Each organoid is a reminder that development is not a one-way street. Cells can be reset, tissues can be coaxed into new forms, and even cognition itself may one day be re-engineered. The beginning is not behind us—it is with us, repeating itself in every culture dish.

Philosophy of Origins

Origins matter because they shape narratives. In mythology, in religion, and in science alike, the story of beginnings frames the story of endings. If organoid intelligence began with a cell, then perhaps its destiny lies in a new definition of what a "mind" can be. The cyclical nature of origins reminds us that progress is rarely linear. Instead, it spirals—returning, reframing, and re-imagining.

By returning to the beginning, we recognize the humility of science. For all our sophistication—microelectrode arrays, CRISPR editing, multimodal profiling—we remain dependent on the most fundamental truth: life emerges from simplicity, from a structure so small it can be seen only under a microscope. To lose sight of this would be to mistake complexity for creation.

12.1 Returning to the Beginning

In the earliest days of stem cell research, the questions were deceptively simple: *Can these cells become neurons? Can they form networks? Could they ever model disease?* Today, after decades of experimentation, those questions have not disappeared; they have only multiplied. The return to the beginning forces us to remember that science is less about answers than about questions that persist and evolve.

An organoid is not valuable because it perfectly mimics the human brain—it does not. Rather, its value lies in its capacity to provoke questions. How much complexity is needed before a system can be called "intelligent"? Does intelligence require consciousness, or is computation enough? Are organoids tools, or do they inch toward becoming participants? These questions echo the very beginnings of philosophy, when human beings first asked what it means to know, to feel, to be. In organoids, the scientific and the philosophical beginnings converge.

Cycles of Innovation

History shows us that every breakthrough is a return disguised as a leap forward. The reprogramming of fibroblasts into iPSCs was not the creation of something entirely new—it was a return to pluripotency, a resetting of fate. The engineering of organoids is similarly a return to development, to embryogenesis played out in miniature. And perhaps the future integration of organoids with artificial intelligence will be a return of another kind: a return to questions about the very nature of mind and machine.

The cyclical nature of innovation means that beginnings are never left behind. They remain embedded in every stage, resurfacing under new names and in new contexts. For organoid intelligence, the beginning is not an origin point in history but an ever-present dynamic, repeating itself in each culture dish and in each philosophical debate.

The Humility of Beginnings

There is a danger in science of forgetting the beginning. As tools become more advanced and results more spectacular, the temptation is to assume mastery. But beginnings remind us that science is not about control but about discovery. No researcher commands a stem cell to self-organize into a neural tube; they merely provide conditions and watch as biology does what it has always done.

To return to the beginning is to return to humility. It is to remember that organoids are not inventions in the way a transistor or algorithm is an invention. They are invitations—opportunities to witness and to learn. If we mistake them for mere tools, we risk reducing life to machinery. If we remember their beginnings, we recognize them as windows into something larger: the resilience and creativity of life itself.

Origins as Destiny

There is a saying that in origins lie destinies. If that is true, then the destiny of organoid intelligence may be bound to the qualities of pluripotency: flexibility, openness, potential without predetermination. Just as pluripotent cells resist fixed fate, so too might organoid intelligence resist being pinned down to a single function or definition. It may evolve in directions we cannot yet imagine, precisely because its beginning is not narrow but expansive.

Returning to the beginning, then, is not nostalgia—it is foresight. It is recognizing that the qualities of origin are seeds of the future. To study organoids is to glimpse what intelligence could be when unbound from the architectures we currently understand.

A Circle, Not a Line

Perhaps the greatest lesson of returning to the beginning is that progress in organoid science is circular, not linear. We began with stem cells, moved into organoids, and now return to questions of identity, ethics, and meaning that are as old as philosophy itself. What has changed is not the question but the context. Where once we debated the soul, we now debate consciousness. Where once we asked whether clay could be given life, we now ask whether silicon and cells together can think.

The circle does not negate progress—it deepens it. Each return to the beginning adds new layers of insight. Each revolution of the circle expands the horizon of possibility.

Conclusion to Section 12.1

Returning to the beginning is not about retracing steps but about realizing that beginnings never leave us. In the story of organoid intelligence, the first cell is always present, pulsing quietly at the heart of every experiment. The future may bring hybrid systems, ethical revolutions, and societal transformations, but all of it is rooted in that moment when science first realized that fate could be rewritten.

As we close this section, we recognize that the story of organoid intelligence is not a straight line into the unknown. It is a spiral, circling back to its beginnings even as it ascends to new heights. And in that spiral lies both humility and hope: humility, because we are reminded of how little we control; hope, because the beginning carries within it infinite possibilities.

12.2 Organoids as Mirrors of Humanity

To gaze at an organoid beneath the microscope is, in a sense, to gaze at ourselves. Though they are only clusters of cells, organoids reflect human identity in profound ways. They mirror not only the biology of our tissues but also the questions we ask about intelligence, creativity, and responsibility. In them, we see both the promise of our science and the shadows of our ambition.

Unlike a silicon chip or a neural network coded in Python, organoids are not wholly products of design. They are living entities, carrying the echoes of billions of years of evolution. When we guide them into forming neural circuits, we are not inventing intelligence from nothing; we are coaxing nature into replaying its own narrative. Thus, organoids are mirrors—not of what we create ex nihilo, but of what we reveal within ourselves.

Biological Reflections

Organoids reflect our biology most directly. Derived from stem cells, they remind us that the human brain itself once began as a simple cluster of proliferating progenitors. In their layers of neurons, their spontaneous firing, and their nascent synaptic networks, we see the processes that once unfolded in our own embryonic development.

The mirror, however, is not perfect. Organoids lack the full architecture of a brain: no blood supply, no sensory inputs, no body to serve. Yet, even in their incompleteness, they reflect a truth we often forget: intelligence is not an all-or-nothing phenomenon. Cognition is not a single leap from silence to thought but a continuum, a gradual orchestration of signals into patterns. In this, organoids mirror the spectrum of intelligence, reminding us that even the most basic networks can carry meaning.

Ethical Reflections

But the mirror extends beyond biology into ethics. When we cultivate organoids, we are confronted by reflections of our own moral choices. What does it mean to nurture a system that may one day approach awareness? Are we caretakers, or are we exploiters? The very existence of organoids pushes us to reflect on how we treat other living beings—animals in laboratories, patients in clinics, even ecosystems on our planet.

Organoids may not yet think, but the mirror they hold forces us to think harder about ourselves. By projecting our hopes and fears onto them, we reveal the ethical contours of our own humanity. In this sense, organoids act less like tools and more like teachers, pushing us toward self-examination.

Philosophical Reflections

Philosophers have long asked: What does it mean to be human? Organoids bring this question into the laboratory. If clusters of cells can fire in coordinated rhythms, if they can process signals and adapt to stimuli, then what separates us from them? Is it scale, complexity, or something intangible we call consciousness?

In these questions, organoids mirror the deepest uncertainties of our species. They challenge the dualisms we have relied upon—human versus machine, natural versus artificial, body versus mind. In their quiet activity, they blur these boundaries, reminding us that identity is not fixed but fluid, shaped as much by perception as by biology.

Organoids as Cultural Mirrors

Beyond science and philosophy, organoids mirror the culture that creates them. In societies enamored with artificial intelligence, organoids embody the desire to merge biology with computation. In cultures anxious about playing God, they reflect the fear of overstepping nature's bounds. The way we talk about organoids—whether as "mini-brains," "living computers," or "ethical dilemmas"—reveals more about us than about them.

12.3 Convergence of Biology, AI, and Philosophy

If the 20th century was the age of physics and computation, the 21st is becoming the age of convergence. Biology no longer sits in isolation from technology, and philosophy no longer lingers only in lecture halls. In the era of organoid intelligence, these three disciplines—biology, artificial intelligence, and philosophy—intertwine in a way that is unprecedented. Each one illuminates the other: biology provides the living substrate, AI provides the tools of analysis and interaction, and philosophy provides the framework to interpret meaning.

This convergence is not accidental. It is driven by necessity. Organoids are too complex to be understood by biology alone, too unpredictable to be guided by technology alone, and too ethically charged to be left without philosophical reflection. To study them is to step into a space where scientific observation, computational power, and human wisdom must co-exist.

Biology: The Living Substrate

At the heart of this convergence is biology. Without stem cells, without organoids, there would be no "living machines." Biology grounds the project in the material reality of life: membranes, ion channels, synapses, and circuits. Each organoid is a condensation of evolutionary history, carrying within it the rules and rhythms that have shaped nervous systems for millions of years.

Yet, biology alone cannot grasp the emergent complexity. To watch neurons fire in organoids is to observe only the surface of a deep ocean. Patterns emerge, but their interpretation requires tools beyond microscopy and electrophysiology. Here AI enters the stage.

Artificial Intelligence: The Analytical Partner

Artificial intelligence acts as both microscope and translator. Neural networks analyze firing patterns, machine learning models classify activity, and predictive algorithms model developmental trajectories. Without AI, the sheer volume of data emerging from organoid experiments would overwhelm human cognition.

But AI is not merely an assistant. It is a collaborator. In learning from organoids, AI itself is reshaped. Traditional machine learning, built on statistical optimization, finds inspiration in the adaptability and plasticity of biological circuits. In turn, organoids can be trained, stimulated, and interfaced with AI systems, forming hybrid loops of information. Biology teaches AI resilience; AI teaches biology interpretation.

Philosophy: The Interpreter

And then comes philosophy, the often-forgotten partner. Organoids force us to ask questions that transcend data: What does it mean for a piece of tissue to process information? At what point does complexity become cognition? Is consciousness an emergent property or an illusion?

Without philosophy, the convergence of biology and AI risks becoming technocratic—powerful but blind. Philosophy anchors the enterprise, reminding us that intelligence is not only about output but also about meaning. It provides the language to grapple with identity, rights, and responsibility.

The Triangle of Convergence

Imagine a triangle: at one corner, biology; at another, AI; at the third, philosophy. Organoid intelligence sits at the center, held in place by the tension and collaboration of all three. Remove one, and the system collapses. With biology alone, we have tissue but no framework. With AI alone, we have algorithms but no embodiment. With philosophy alone, we have speculation but no experiment. Together, they form a new paradigm—one where life, computation, and meaning converge.

Toward a New Epistemology

This convergence also heralds a new way of knowing. Traditional science sought objectivity by stripping away values; traditional philosophy sought meaning by stepping outside of experiment; traditional AI sought efficiency by ignoring context. In organoid intelligence, none of these approaches is sufficient in isolation. What emerges is a new epistemology: knowledge as collaboration.

In this model, the laboratory is not just a place of experiments but a dialogue between disciplines. Data is interpreted through algorithms, algorithms are questioned by philosophy, and philosophy is grounded again in biology. Truth is no longer a product of one method but of convergence itself.

12.4 Ethical Horizons and Bio-Rights

Every frontier of science eventually collides with the frontier of ethics. For organoid intelligence, that collision is not in the distant future—it is already here. When clusters of human-derived cells begin to organize, to signal, and to respond, the old categories of "tool" and "subject" blur. Are organoids merely experimental models, or do they possess the beginnings of something we would recognize as moral status? Do they belong to the same ethical landscape as laboratory animals, or do they demand an entirely new framework of rights?

This section explores the ethical horizons of organoid intelligence: the dilemmas, the philosophical debates, and the concept of bio-rights—the idea that living systems, even if subhuman or pre-conscious, may deserve recognition within our moral and legal systems.

The Threshold of Moral Consideration

Ethics often revolves around thresholds. A zygote becomes an embryo; an embryo becomes a fetus; at some point, a fetus is granted rights. Animals are accorded different moral statuses based on their perceived capacity for suffering or cognition. Organoids complicate this logic. They are not full brains, yet they exhibit neural firing patterns. They do not experience pain as animals do, yet they process information in ways that are undeniably brain-like.

Where, then, is the threshold? At what point does a cluster of cells merit moral consideration? Some argue that without sensory input, organoids cannot suffer and thus fall outside the ethical circle. Others counter that the potential for cognitive complexity itself is enough to warrant caution. In this uncertainty lies the urgency of the debate.

Lessons from Animal Ethics

The history of animal research offers both guidance and warning. For centuries, animals were treated as mere instruments. Only in recent decades have legal frameworks recognized their capacity for suffering, leading to regulations on humane treatment and alternatives to animal use. Organoids may follow a similar trajectory, moving from instruments to entities deserving of ethical safeguards.

But the analogy is imperfect. Organoids lack bodies, instincts, and evolutionary histories. They are not animals miniaturized, but emergent systems whose status is ambiguous. This ambiguity makes them ethically unprecedented.

Bio-Rights: A New Frontier

The concept of **bio-rights** emerges from this ambiguity. Bio-rights suggest that living systems—whether organoids, synthetic embryos, or other biohybrids—may deserve recognition not because they are human, but because they embody capacities that challenge our moral categories.

Bio-rights need not imply full human rights. They may instead involve guidelines for cultivation, limits on experimentation, and obligations of transparency. Just as international law restricts human cloning, so too might future frameworks restrict certain manipulations of organoids. The point is not to anthropomorphize them but to acknowledge that their existence provokes responsibility.

The Slippery Slope Concern

Critics warn of a slippery slope: grant organoids rights, and where does it end? Would every tissue sample gain protection? Would research grind to a halt under excessive caution? The counterargument is that ignoring bio-rights risks an even steeper slope—one toward exploitation without reflection, where living systems are instrumentalized without restraint.

Ethics, in this view, is not a brake on science but a compass. It does not halt progress but guides it toward outcomes that respect both discovery and dignity.

Toward Global Frameworks

Already, international organizations such as the ISSCR (International Society for Stem Cell Research) are drafting guidelines for organoid research. Yet these remain fragmented and advisory. What is needed is a global framework, akin to the bioethics declarations of UNESCO or the treaties on genetic editing. Such frameworks would recognize the unique status of organoids: not mere tissue, not full beings, but something in between.

A global conversation is essential because organoids cross borders. What one country bans, another may permit. Without coordination, ethical tourism may emerge, where experiments migrate to the most permissive jurisdictions. A unified framework would prevent such disparities and foster trust in the legitimacy of the field.

Conclusion

The ethical horizons of organoid intelligence are vast and unsettled. Bio-rights may one day become a cornerstone of law and policy, reshaping how we view life in all its forms. For now, they serve as a reminder: that science cannot advance without reflection, that progress without responsibility is regression, and that in the mirror of organoids we confront not only biology but the essence of our humanity.

12.5 Futures Within Reach: 5, 10, 30, 50 Years

The story of organoid intelligence is not confined to the present. Its true significance lies in its potential to reshape the decades ahead. Unlike many scientific tools, organoids are not incremental—they are generative. They do not simply extend existing technologies; they redefine what technology can mean. To glimpse the future of organoid intelligence, we must imagine a timeline: not a prophecy, but a map of plausible horizons. In this section, we sketch the possibilities of the next 5, 10, 30, and 50 years, acknowledging that each horizon carries both promise and peril.

The Next 5 Years: Consolidation and Standardization

The immediate horizon is one of refinement. In the next five years, organoid science will likely focus on standardization, reproducibility, and scalability. Today, no two organoids are exactly alike, making experiments difficult to compare across laboratories. The challenge of reproducibility has already sparked initiatives to develop standardized protocols, biomimetic scaffolds, and controlled bioreactors.

We can expect:

- Reliable brain organoid protocols that yield predictable architectures.
- Integration with high-throughput screening for drug discovery, enabling pharmaceutical companies to test compounds on hundreds of patient-derived organoids simultaneously.
- Stronger ethical guidelines as public awareness grows. Early frameworks for bio-rights may begin to take shape, especially in Europe and North America.
- Early AI integration: neural activity from organoids will be processed by machine learning pipelines, creating initial biohybrid models for signal classification.

In this horizon, organoids remain laboratory phenomena. Their impact is felt most in medicine and basic neuroscience, not yet in society at large.

The Next 10 Years: Organoids in Precision Medicine

By a decade from now, organoids will likely transition from research tools to clinical companions. Personalized medicine, once a buzzword, may become reality through patient-derived organoids.

We can envision:

- Patient avatars: a cancer patient's tumor organoid tested against dozens of therapies to predict the most effective treatment.
- Neurological disease modeling: Alzheimer's, Parkinson's, and ALS organoids used to screen experimental drugs.
- Hybrid diagnostics: AI trained on thousands of organoid responses, offering predictive analytics for clinicians.
- Public debate: ethical questions surrounding organoids may enter mainstream culture, especially if neural organoids begin to display unexpected complexity.

In this horizon, organoids enter hospitals and clinics, becoming extensions of the patient, partners in decision-making, and tools for reducing trial-and-error medicine.

The Next 30 Years: Hybrid Cognition

Three decades from now, the boundaries between organoids and machines may blur. Organoid intelligence could evolve from model systems into biohybrid processors—living networks integrated with silicon.

Possible milestones include:

- Bio-computational platforms: organoids embedded in chips, processing signals in ways silicon alone cannot replicate.
- Adaptive AI: machine learning algorithms inspired by organoid plasticity, capable of continual learning without catastrophic forgetting.
- Neural symbiosis: organoids trained to interact with sensors, controlling robotic limbs or navigating digital environments.
- Philosophical reckoning: if organoids exhibit emergent properties resembling learning or memory, society will confront whether these systems are simply tools or something more.

By this stage, organoids may no longer be confined to laboratories or clinics. They may inhabit devices, research centers, even computational infrastructures. The question will not be whether organoids are intelligent, but how their intelligence differs from—and complements—our own.

The Next 50 Years: A New Epoch of Intelligence

Half a century from now, organoid intelligence could represent a turning point in human history. Just as the transistor defined the 20th century, biohybrid intelligence may define the 21st.

We can imagine:

- Global bio-computing networks: organoid-based processors distributed across the planet, contributing to climate modeling, medical research, and even space exploration.
- Consciousness debates: if organoids reach thresholds of complexity indistinguishable from rudimentary consciousness, humanity may face unprecedented ethical and legal questions.
- Post-human collaboration: organoids may no longer be "tools" but "partners," co-authors of knowledge, co-navigators of discovery.
- Interplanetary applications: organoid-AI hybrids deployed in space, where their adaptability makes them more resilient than silicon in extreme environments.

The 50-year horizon is speculative, but speculation is itself a form of preparation. To imagine is to prepare for the responsibilities such futures demand.

Conclusion

Mapping the future of organoid intelligence is not an exercise in fantasy but in foresight. The next five decades may transform organoids from fragile clusters of cells into central actors in science, medicine, and society. Each horizon—5, 10, 30, 50 years—represents not only progress but responsibility. What we choose today will echo into futures we may never live to see.

Organoids remind us that beginnings are eternal, but so too are futures. To return to the beginning is to glimpse the seed; to look to the horizon is to see the forest yet to grow.

12.6 Society and the Bio-Economy

Science does not exist in isolation. Every discovery ripples outward, reshaping society and its institutions. The emergence of organoid intelligence promises not only to advance laboratories and clinics but also to transform economies, redefine industries, and challenge cultural norms. In this section, we explore how society might adapt to the rise of organoid intelligence and how a new **bio-economy**—an economy driven not by silicon alone but by living intelligence—may emerge.

Education and Research Institutions

Universities will be among the first to feel the impact. Just as computer science departments reshaped campuses in the late 20th century, departments of organoid intelligence and biohybrid systems may arise in the 21st. Students will not only learn biology and engineering but also ethics, law, and philosophy as integral components of their training.

Research institutions may pivot toward interdisciplinary centers where biologists, AI specialists, ethicists, and entrepreneurs collaborate. The division between natural sciences and humanities may blur as the study of organoids demands both technical skill and philosophical insight. Education itself will be reshaped, producing not only scientists but also custodians of a new form of intelligence.

Healthcare Transformation

Medicine will undergo perhaps the most immediate transformation. Organoid models already promise breakthroughs in drug testing and personalized therapies. As these practices become mainstream, healthcare systems may shift from reactive to proactive, from generalized treatments to individualized strategies.

- Hospitals may establish "organoid clinics," where patient-derived mini-brains or mini-hearts are maintained for ongoing diagnostic testing.
- Insurance companies may incorporate organoid data into coverage decisions, offering policies tailored to the predictive models derived from biohybrid analytics.
- Pharmaceutical industries may save billions by screening drugs on organoid panels before entering costly clinical trials.

Healthcare costs may decrease, but new inequalities may arise: who will have access to personalized organoid diagnostics? Will wealthier nations monopolize the benefits, leaving poorer regions behind?

Industry and Technology

The bio-economy extends beyond healthcare. Tech companies may integrate organoid processors into computational devices. Unlike silicon chips, organoids offer adaptability and learning in real time. A future smartphone could contain not just circuits but living networks capable of context-sensitive reasoning.

New industries will arise:

- Bioreactor manufacturing for large-scale cultivation of organoids.
- Data integration companies specializing in translating biological signals into computational code.
- Ethics and compliance firms ensuring adherence to international bio-rights frameworks.

The convergence of biology and computation may produce an economic boom reminiscent of the digital revolution, but grounded in living systems rather than binary code.

Cultural Impact

Culture will not remain untouched. Just as AI sparked debates about art, authorship, and creativity, organoid intelligence will provoke questions about identity and meaning. If organoids can compose music, solve problems, or assist in research, are they collaborators or tools? Cultural narratives—films, novels, art—will grapple with these questions, shaping public perception.

Religion and philosophy may also respond. Some traditions may view organoid intelligence as overstepping human boundaries, while others may see it as an extension of human creativity bestowed by evolution or divinity. Public opinion will oscillate between fascination and fear, admiration and resistance.

Economic Inequalities and Global Access

The rise of the bio-economy will magnify global disparities unless deliberate efforts are made to ensure access. Wealthy nations with advanced research infrastructure will accelerate ahead, creating new forms of technological dominance. Developing countries may become dependent on imported biohybrid technologies, deepening existing inequalities.

A fair bio-economy will require international cooperation:

- Shared databases of organoid research accessible to all.
- Global funding initiatives to support labs in low-income countries.
- Ethical trade policies preventing exploitation of biological resources.

The alternative is a world where the benefits of organoid intelligence concentrate in a few regions, exacerbating divides rather than bridging them.

Toward a Living Economy

Unlike the digital economy, which thrives on data, the bio-economy thrives on life itself. This raises profound questions: what does it mean to commodify living systems? Is an organoid processor a product, a partner, or something in between?

A living economy challenges us to rethink value. Profit cannot be the sole measure when the resources at stake are semi-living, semi-cognitive systems. The bio-economy must balance innovation with responsibility, growth with guardianship. If done wisely, it could become not only profitable but also regenerative, aligning human progress with the principles of life itself.

Conclusion

Society and the bio-economy will be transformed by organoid intelligence. Universities, hospitals, industries, and cultures will all be reshaped. New opportunities will arise, but so will inequalities. The challenge is not only to innovate but also to distribute fairly, not only to create but also to care.

In the mirror of organoids, society sees both its ambition and its fragility. The bio-economy could either replicate the inequities of the past or pioneer a more inclusive future. The choice, as always, is ours.

12.7 A Message to the Next Generation

Every book is, in some sense, a letter to the future. The chapters you have read so far are not only about what organoid intelligence is today, but what it may become in the hands of those who will continue this journey. This section is written directly to you—the students, the researchers, the dreamers, and the skeptics who will shape the decades ahead.

The Torch of Curiosity

Science is not inherited like property; it is inherited like fire. Each generation receives the flame of curiosity, not the ashes of old knowledge. Organoid intelligence is still in its infancy, and its trajectory depends not on what has been discovered, but on what will be pursued with imagination and courage.

To the next generation: you are the torchbearers. You will decide whether organoids remain laboratory curiosities or evolve into transformative partners of humanity. Your curiosity is not trivial; it is destiny.

The Burden of Responsibility

With curiosity comes responsibility. Organoids are not like microscopes or test tubes—they are living systems, carrying the potential for cognitive processes. To work with them is to engage in a dialogue with life itself. The choices you make—what to study, what to publish, what to withhold—will reverberate through ethics, culture, and policy.

The next generation must resist the temptation to see organoids merely as tools. You must treat them as mirrors that reflect your own values. Ask yourself not only "What can I do?" but "What should I do?" The burden of responsibility is heavy, but it is also a sign of maturity—the maturity of science, and the maturity of humanity.

Innovation Beyond Boundaries

You will inherit a world of convergence, where biology, AI, and philosophy intertwine. Do not be afraid to cross boundaries. The greatest breakthroughs will not come from staying within disciplines but from weaving them together. The next Darwin may also need to understand machine learning; the next Turing may also need to grapple with bioethics.

Your generation has the opportunity to redefine what it means to be a scientist, a philosopher, an engineer. Do not let old divisions confine you. Innovation belongs to those who dare to imagine connections where others see walls.

The Human Dimension

Remember that science is not only about data; it is about people. Patients waiting for treatments, societies wrestling with new technologies, cultures seeking meaning—all of them are part of the story of organoid intelligence. If you pursue this field, do so with empathy. Listen not only to neurons firing in a dish but also to the voices of those who will be affected by your work.

The future you build must not be only powerful but also humane. In your hands lies the possibility of aligning discovery with dignity.

A Call to Courage

Progress requires courage: the courage to ask questions that unsettle, to face uncertainty, to admit ignorance, and to take responsibility for consequences. Organoid intelligence will present challenges that no textbook has prepared you for. You may face dilemmas without clear answers, pressures from industries and governments, and fears from the public.

Do not retreat. Face these challenges with honesty and humility. Courage is not arrogance; it is the willingness to move forward even when the path is unclear.

Conclusion: The Story Continues

The message to the next generation is simple: the story of organoid intelligence is now your story. You inherit its promises and its perils, its questions and its possibilities. The flame is in your hands.

If there is one truth that echoes across time, it is this: beginnings never end. Each generation returns to the beginning, reinterprets it, and carries it forward. So too will you.

May your work honor the origins, expand the horizons, and write the next chapter in the story of life and intelligence.

12.8 Closing Reflections

Every journey must end, but endings are also beginnings in disguise. As we close this book, we stand at a threshold—not of finality, but of possibility. The story of organoid intelligence is far from finished; indeed, it has barely begun. What we have explored in these chapters is not a destination but a map, a compass pointing toward horizons that stretch beyond our sight.

From a Single Cell to Infinite Horizons

It began with a single cell, pluripotent and undefined. From that cell, organoids emerged—clusters of life that recapitulate the earliest chapters of our own existence. In their formation, we rediscovered the power of self-organization, the elegance of simplicity giving rise to complexity.

Step by step, we followed the story:

- The genesis of stem cells.
- The building of mini-brains.
- The listening of neural circuits.
- The editing of blueprints through CRISPR.
- The profiling of omics.
- The integration with artificial intelligence.
- The reckoning with ethics.
- The anticipation of futures.

Each chapter was not a conclusion, but a piece of a spiral that always returns to its origin, even as it ascends higher.

The Mirror and the Horizon

Organoids have become our mirrors, reflecting our creativity, our fears, and our responsibilities. They remind us that intelligence is not unique to scale or species; it is a property of systems capable of adaptation and self-organization. In them, we see ourselves—not in full, but in fragments, as though gazing at a reflection in water, rippling and incomplete.

But they also point us toward the horizon. They whisper of futures in which biology and computation coalesce, in which medicine becomes personal, in which ethics must expand to include new forms of life. The horizon is vast, unfinished, and uncertain. Yet it is there that meaning resides—not in final answers, but in enduring questions.

Science as Responsibility

The closing reflection must also be a reminder: science is not neutral. Every experiment carries within it a choice. To cultivate organoids without reflection would be to wield power without wisdom. To refuse the challenge out of fear would be to abandon possibility. The path forward lies in balance—in cultivating both discovery and dignity, both progress and humility.

Organoid intelligence is not just about what we can build; it is about what kind of world we choose to inhabit. The question is not only whether organoids can think, but whether we can think wisely about organoids.

An Invitation

This book ends, but the story does not. The next chapters will be written by those who enter laboratories, who code algorithms, who draft ethical frameworks, who imagine futures. To you, the reader, this is not only information but an invitation. The horizon awaits, and you are part of its unfolding.

Closing Words

The tale of organoid intelligence is the tale of life returning to itself: cells that reflect minds, minds that reflect cells. We began at the beginning; we end at the horizon. Yet even as we close, the spiral continues, carrying us forward.

"The horizon of organoid intelligence is not the end of the story—it is the beginning of a new chapter in the story of life itself."

References

1. Lancaster MA, Knoblich JA. Organogenesis in a dish: Modeling development and disease using organoid technologies. Science. 2014;345(6194):1247125.

2. Quadrato G, Brown J, Arlotta P. The promises and challenges of human brain organoids as models of neuropsychiatric disease. Nat Med. 2016;22(11):1220–1228.

3. Yamanaka S. Strategies and new developments in the generation of patient-specific pluripotent stem cells. Cell Stem Cell. 2007;1(1):39–49.

4. Kelava I, Lancaster MA. Stem cell models of human brain development. Cell Stem Cell. 2016;18(6):736–748.

5. Clevers H. Modeling development and disease with organoids. Cell. 2016;165(7):1586–1597.

6. Trujillo CA, Muotri AR. Brain organoids and the study of neurodevelopment. Trends Mol Med. 2018;24(12):982–990.

7. Mansour AA, Gonçalves JT, Bloyd CW, Li H, Fernandes S, Quang D, et al. An in vivo model of functional and vascularized human brain organoids. Nat Biotechnol. 2018;36(5):432–441.

8. Smirnova L, Caffo BS, Gracias DH, Harris G, Hengstler JG, Hoeng J, et al. Organoid intelligence (OI): The new frontier in biocomputing and biohybrid intelligence. Front Sci. 2023;1:1–19.

9. Paşca AM, Sloan SA, Clarke LE, Tian Y, Makinson CD, Huber N, et al. Functional cortical

neurons and astrocytes from human pluripotent stem cells in 3D culture. Nat Methods. 2015;12(7):671–678.

10. Bhaduri A, Andrews MG, Mancia Leon W, Jung D, Shin D, Allen D, et al. Cell stress in cortical organoids impairs molecular subtype specification. Nature. 2020;578:142–148.

11. Kanton S, Boyle MJ, He Z, Santel M, Weigert A, Sanchís-Calleja F, et al. Organoid single-cell genomic atlas uncovers human-specific features of brain development. Nature. 2019;574:418–422.

12. Quadrato G, Nguyen T, Macosko E, Sherwood J, Yang S, Berger D, et al. Cell diversity and network dynamics in photosensitive human brain organoids. Nature. 2017;545:48–53.

13. Camp JG, Badsha F, Florio M, Kanton S, Gerber T, Wilsch-Bräuninger M, et al. Human cerebral organoids recapitulate gene expression programs of fetal neocortex development. Proc Natl Acad Sci U S A. 2015;112(51):15672–15677.

14. Jo J, Xiao Y, Sun AX, Cukuroglu E, Tran HD, Göke J, et al. Midbrain-like organoids from human pluripotent stem cells contain functional dopaminergic and neuromelanin-producing neurons. Cell Stem Cell. 2016;19(2):248–257.

15. Di Lullo E, Kriegstein AR. The use of brain organoids to investigate neural development and disease. Nat Rev Neurosci. 2017;18(9):573–584.

16. Sloan SA, Darmanis S, Huber N, Khan TA, Birey F, Caneda C, et al. Human astrocyte maturation captured in 3D cerebral cortical spheroids derived from pluripotent stem cells. Neuron. 2017;95(4):779–790.

17.Velasco S, Kedaigle AJ, Simmons SK, Nash A, Rocha M, Quadrato G, et al. Individual brain organoids reproducibly form cell diversity of the human cerebral cortex. Nature. 2019;570:523–527.

18.Fair SR, Julian D, Hartlaub AM, Pusuluri ST, Malik G, Summerfied TL, et al. Electrophysiological maturation of cerebral organoids correlates with dynamic morphological and cellular development. Stem Cell Reports. 2020;15(4):855–868.

19.Qian X, Song H, Ming GL. Brain organoids: Advances, applications and challenges. Development. 2019;146(8):dev166074.

20.Muotri AR. The human model: Changing focus on autism research. Biol Psychiatry. 2019;85(4):269–276.

21.Schwartz MP, Hou Z, Propson NE, Zhang J, Engstrom CJ, Costa VS, et al. Human pluripotent stem cell-derived neural constructs for predicting neural toxicity. Proc Natl Acad Sci U S A. 2015;112(40):12516–12521.

22.Quadrato G, Arlotta P. Present and future of modeling human brain development in 3D organoids. Curr Opin Cell Biol. 2017;49:47–52.

23.Sharf T, van der Molen T, Guzman E, Chandrasekaran S, Maffioletti SM, et al. Data-driven reconstruction of regulatory networks in human brain organoids. Cell Stem Cell. 2021;28(1):56–72.

24.Lancaster MA, Renner M, Martin CA, Wenzel D, Bicknell LS, Hurles ME, et al. Cerebral organoids model human brain development and microcephaly. Nature. 2013;501:373–379.

25.Pollen AA, Bhaduri A, Andrews MG, Nowakowski TJ, Meyerson OS, Mostajo-Radji MA, et al. Establishing cerebral organoids as models of human-specific brain evolution. Cell. 2019;176(4):743–756.

26.Fiddes IT, Lodewijk GA, Mooring M, Bosworth CM, Ewing AD, Mantalas GL, et al. Human-specific NOTCH2NL genes affect notch signaling and cortical neurogenesis. Cell. 2018;173(6):1356–1369.

27.Giandomenico SL, Mierau SB, Gibbons GM, Wenger LM, Masullo L, Sit T, et al. Cerebral organoids at the air–liquid interface generate diverse nerve tracts with functional output. Nat Neurosci. 2019;22:669–679.

28.Quadrato G, Arlotta P. Technologies for the study of 3D brain organoids. Nat Biotechnol. 2017;35(9):833–851.

29.Shou Y, Liang F, Xu S, Li X. The application of brain organoids: From basic research to translational medicine. J Biomed Sci. 2020;27:25.

30.Costamagna G, Comi GP, Corti S. Advancing drug discovery for neurological disorders using iPSC-derived neural organoids. Int J Mol Sci. 2021;22(2):976.

31.Park J, Wetzel I, Marriott I, Dréau D, D'Avanzo C, Kim DY, et al. A 3D human triculture system modeling neurodegeneration and neuroinflammation. Nat Neurosci. 2018;21:941–951.

32.Pamies D, Barreras P, Block K, Makri G, Kumar A, Wiersma D, et al. A human brain microphysiological system derived from induced pluripotent stem cells to study neurological diseases. ALTEX. 2017;34(3):362–376.

33.Amin ND, Paşca SP. Building models of brain disorders with three-dimensional organoids. Neuron. 2018;100(2):389–405.

34.Birey F, Andersen J, Makinson CD, Islam S, Wei W, Huber N, et al. Assembly of functionally integrated human forebrain spheroids. Nature. 2017;545:54–59.

35.Kim H, Park HJ, Choi H, Chang Y, Park H, Shin J, et al. Modeling GBA1-associated Parkinson's disease using patient-derived midbrain organoids. Sci Transl Med. 2019;11(472):eaax1768.

36.Raja WK, Mungenast AE, Lin YT, Ko T, Abdurrob F, Seo J, et al. Self-organizing 3D human neural tissue derived from induced pluripotent stem cells recapitulates Alzheimer's disease phenotypes. PLoS One. 2016;11(9):e0161969.

37.Choi SH, Kim YH, Hebisch M, Sliwinski C, Lee S, D'Avanzo C, et al. A three-dimensional human neural cell culture model of Alzheimer's disease. Nature. 2014;515:274–278.

38.Gordon A, Yoon SJ, Tran SS, Makinson CD, Park JY, Andersen J, et al. Long-term maturation of human cortical organoids matches key early postnatal transitions. Nat Neurosci. 2021;24:331–342.

39.Gabriel E, Gopalakrishnan J. Generation of iPSC-derived human brain organoids: An overview. Biol Psychiatry. 2017;82(5):375–385.

40.Eura N, Matsui T, Luginbühl J, Matsubayashi M, Matsuda M, Ebisuya M. Brain organoids recapitulate the spatiotemporal pattern of early neurodevelopment. Nat Commun. 2020;11:5140.

41.Cugola FR, Fernandes IR, Russo FB, Freitas BC, Dias JLM, Guimarães KP, et al. The Brazilian Zika virus strain causes birth defects in experimental models. Nature. 2016;534:267–271.

42.Watanabe M, Buth JE, Vishlaghi N, de la Torre-Ubieta L, Taxidis J, Khakh BS, et al. Self-organized cerebral organoids with human-specific features predict effective drugs to combat Zika virus infection. Cell Reports. 2017;21(2):517–532.

43.Monzel AS, Smits LM, Hemmer K, Hachi S, Moreno EL, van Wuellen T, et al. Derivation of human midbrain-specific organoids from neuroepithelial stem cells. Stem Cell Reports. 2017;8(5):1144–1154.

44.Renner M, Lancaster MA, Bian S, Choi H, Ku T, Peer A, et al. Self-patterned human organoids with integrated brain regions. Nature. 2017;545:48–53.

45.Trujillo CA, Gao R, Negraes PD, Gu J, Buchanan J, Preissl S, et al. Complex oscillatory waves emerging from cortical organoids model early human brain network development. Cell Stem Cell. 2019;25(4):558–569.

46.Miura Y, Li MY, Birey F, Ikeda K, Revah O, Thete MV, et al. Generation of human striatal organoids and cortico-striatal assembloids from human pluripotent stem cells. Nat Biotechnol. 2020;38(12):1421–1430.

47.Xiang Y, Tanaka Y, Patterson B, Kang YJ, Govindaiah G, Roselaar N, et al. Fusion of regionally specified hPSC-derived organoids models human brain development and interneuron migration. Cell Stem Cell. 2017;21(3):383–398.

48.Birey F, Andersen J, Paşca SP. Assembly of regionally specified brain organoids. Nat Protoc. 2021;16(6):2739–2763.

49.Chen HI, Song H, Ming GL. Applications of human brain organoids to clinical problems. Dev Dyn. 2019;248(1):53–64.

50.Quadrato G, Arlotta P. Ethical considerations of brain organoid research. Curr Opin Neurobiol. 2020;61:102–110.

51.Farahany NA, Greely HT, Hurlbut JB, Lunshof JE, Scott CT, Jabr F, et al. The ethics of experimenting with human brain tissue. Nature. 2018;556:429–432.

52.Lavazza A, Massimini M. Cerebral organoids: Ethical issues and consciousness assessment. Stem Cell Reports. 2018;10(2):335–341.

53.Muotri AR. Organoid intelligence (OI): Challenges and opportunities of connecting stem cell-derived brains to machines. Trends Neurosci. 2021;44(9):699–711.

Acknowledgments

This book was not written in isolation; it is the result of many quiet acts of love, guidance, and encouragement.

First and foremost, I thank my parents, whose unwavering support and endless patience became the ground on which all my efforts stood. Their strength was my compass, their love my foundation.

To my brother, my companion in both silence and laughter, thank you for being a constant source of encouragement and light. Your presence has been like a lighthouse guiding me through uncertain seas.

To my colleagues and students, your curiosity and critical reflections sharpened my vision and gave this work its true vitality.

And finally, to every reader who holds this book in their hands: it is in your curiosity that these pages find meaning. Without you, the story of organoid intelligence would remain unfinished.

About the Author

Mahdi Yousefian is a researcher and writer fascinated by the intersection of biology, technology, and philosophy.

His work focuses on organoid intelligence—tiny, self-organizing systems that may one day reshape our understanding of both the human brain and the future of artificial intelligence.

With a background in life sciences and a passion for multidisciplinary inquiry, he bridges the worlds of laboratory research and philosophical reflection. His goal is not only to explain how science works, but to ask what it means—for humanity, for society, and for the generations to come.

When not immersed in research or writing, he finds joy in reading across diverse fields, exploring ethical questions in science, and sharing knowledge with curious minds.

This book, "Organoid Intelligence: The Dawn of Living Machines", is his first major work, written with the hope of inspiring wonder and dialogue about the new horizons where biology meets technology.

www.ingramcontent.com/pod-product-compliance
Lightning Source LLC
LaVergne TN
LVHW010728090726
842905LV00040B/963
9798232626945